7 MINUTES TO CLARITY ACTIVITY BOOK

WHAT IS MINDFULNESS?

When you think of mindfulness, what comes to your mind first? Is it a definition, an opinion, a perception or a belief? According to Merriam-Webster Dictionary, Mindfulness is: "the practice of maintaining a non-judgmental state of heightened or complete awareness of one's thoughts, emotions, or experiences on a moment-to-moment basis."

The common meaning would be "being mindful, conscious or aware about something". But, Mindfulness in the context here would be solely regarding the state of our mind- the quality of our mental space.

Mindfulness means keeping up with our thoughts, feelings, bodily sensations and our environment by tuning our senses to focus on the present rather than the past or future. It is the state of awareness we take in, control and acknowledge when we allow ourselves to experience the beauty in the present moments around us. We tend to get caught up in too many things that either drag us back to the past or make us stuck in the future we imagine. As a result, we unconsciously or consciously ignore the power of the present and instead, we get lost in the voices inside our heads. When we become mindful of these things, our reason, values and purpose in life becomes rekindled.

The American Psychological Association (APA.org, 2012) defines Mindfulness as:

"…a moment-to-moment awareness of one's experience without judgment. In this sense, mindfulness is a state and not a trait. While it might be promoted by certain practices or activities, such as meditation, it is not equivalent to or synonymous with them."

Jon Kabat Zinn, who is significantly recognised globally for his work on mindfulness-based stress reduction (MBSR) also defines mindfulness as:

"The awareness that arises from paying attention, on purpose, in the present moment and non-judgmentally" (Kabat-Zinn, in Purser, 2015).

Mindfulness is known to originate from Buddhist meditation, the renowned and profane practice of mindfulness. However, it became a trend after the work of Jon Kabat-Zinn and the Mindfulness-Based Stress Reduction (MBSR) program, which he launched in Massachusetts Medical School in 1979. Since then, thousands of studies have documented the physical and mental health benefits of mindfulness in general and MBSR in particular, inspiring countless programs to adapt the MBSR model for a wide variety of contexts like schools, prisons, hospitals, workplaces and beyond.

There is really no main definition or streamlined group of definitions for Mindfulness. Mindfulness can be described, explained, portrayed and embodied in different ways. Hence, based on the various definitions dedicated to this concept, there are things you should know. These things shape the context of Mindfulness as a whole; which is why we need to know them before we can benefit from Mindfulness as a lifestyle.

1). Mindfulness is the reverseof Mindlessness

Do you ever get so carried away by what you intend to do for the day, and you just realise that you didn't even notice when time had pass? Have you ever gone out to actually do something, and then you forget what you actually intended to do? When these things happen, we loose track of events around us. The things that seemed easy to place our attention to becomes more difficult day by day. This is what is called mindlessness.

Unlike mindlessness, mindfulness occurs when we are in control of our attention span. It involves us deliberately shifting our attention to things without judging ourselves. Mindfulness prevents you from loosing yourself to harmful effects of mindlessness. Learning to be mindful wakes us up from that autopilot or sleepwalking mode and switches off those suffocating voices in our heads. It allows us to actually live the life we need-based a peaceful, calm life free from wander, anxiety, depression, absent mindedness and so on.

Both concepts completely differ from each other, but yet they tend to be underemphasized. Mindlessness denotes close-handedness in the way of handling information and situations, while Mindfulness is totally open-handedness to these things. The former is a lack of conscious awareness by virtue of little attention and commitment to detail, while the latter is the complete opposite.

2). Mindfulness is self-regulating

One uncommon feature of this concept that you should know is that it helps you regulate where you put your attention at. When you can manage the way you you shift attention to things, then you can regulate your concentration game. With this feature, mindfulness exposes you to an attitude of curiosity, acceptance and openness.

Self-regulation of attention increases recognition of mental events in the present moments. With self-regulation, we subconsciously adopt a particular orientation towards our experiences in the present moment- an orientation that is characterized by curiosity, openness, and acceptance.

3). Mindfulness is not to be taken with levity

Daniel J. Siegel states that; "Mindfulness in its most general sense is about waking up from a life on automatic, and being sensitive to novelty in our everyday experiences . . . Instead of being on automatic and mindless, mindfulness helps us awaken, and by reflecting on the mind we are enabled to make choices and thus change becomes possible" (Hampton, 2014).

Our sensitivity deploys from our emotions, therefore our emotions should not be treated insensitively. The ability for us to make it an habit of appreciating the little things that occur moments-by-momemts, the acceptance we build in us as a sense of alertness without being judgemental and the way we choose to stream down our thoughts and feelings to the beauty of the present all comes down to the capacity of our emotions.

Mindfulness is not just about regarding only the things we should view as important, but it is also about opening up the whole of our emotions, and allowing them flow with these mind-habits. It conveys us to times in our lives where we can approach our experiences and unleash our minds with caring, kindness and warmth to ourselves and to others. Thich Nhat Hanh said the same thing when saying that:

"Mindfulness shows us what is happening in our bodies, our emotions, our minds, and in the world. Through mindfulness, we avoid harming ourselves and others."

Mindfulness comes by belief. When we believe, we demonstrate proof of its positive effects in every aspect of our lives, including our health, career, family and other relationships.

4). Mindfulness means to return to the present moment.

Mindfulness is about staying present in the moment and observing what happens at that present moment, instead of allowing those moments to wander away in our thoughts. Our minds if left alone, can remain engaged in replaying the past or imagining the future non-stop. Now, this is where people get mistaken. Mindfulness does not mean the possibility of staying in the present moments is 100% guaranteed. There are times that our minds would tend to naturally slip away into the past, future or tension around us currently. That is just reality and it is normal. What makes us mindful is when we have that power to control our minds to return back to the beauty of the present moments. When we learn to be mindful, we have control over our mind, and we can therefore, distinguish between we getting caught up in our heads and we actually immersing our attention in the present.

Staying at the present moment also implies that we remain there without being overwhelmed or overly reactive to what is right or wrong and what goes on around us. It involves us being fully present.

5). Mindfulness is all about being deliberate

Being deliberate also means being intentional, being aware, being observant and being conscious. It means going things on purpose. Regardless of whatever synonym is used here, Mindfulness evolves around the deliberate direction of our attention. Being mindful portrays that we step into the conscious lifestyle. We become more awake and step up from that dormant mode where our thought process was to an aware, balanced acceptance of the present experience.

Sharon Salzberg said that: "Mindfulness isn't just about knowing that you are hearing something, seeing something, or even observing that you're having a particular feeling. It's about doing so in a certain way—with balance and equanimity, and without judgment. Mindfulness is the practice of paying attention in a way that creates space for insight" (2015).

When we are deliberate, we perceive things without constriction; with all the senses in our body from the taste in our mouth to the feel of air on our faces. Mindfulness makes us recognise that we are more than our thoughts or feelings. In as much as we possess the natural ability to be aware of our thoughts, feelings, sounds, how our body feels, the environment etc., we are not driven by these. We take a step back and observe reality just as it is, no more, no less. We see our mind's habit of creating stories about how reality should be that make us suffer when our expectations are not met. When we are mindful, we suspend reactivity and begin to see and accept reality as it is.

6). Mindfulness requires practice and training

Mindfulness is not some special thing we do. We already have the innate capacity to be present, and it doesn't require us to change who we are. But we can cultivate these innate qualities with simple meditation practices that are scientifically demonstrated to benefit ourselves, our loved ones, our friends and neighbors, the people we work with, and the institutions and organizations we take part in.

Mindfulness is activated with consistent practice. You need to train yourself to do things in a specific way. If you are training yourself or a person is mindful, it must align with the following:

(1) Try not to think about anything that went on in the past or that might be coming up in future

(2) Always pay attention to what's going on around. Concentrate on them with purpose

(3) Focus on the present moment

(4) Learn to be non-judgemental about anything noticed. Do not label things as 'good' or 'bad'"

7). Mindfulness makes us better versions of ourselves

No matter how far we think we've drifted apart, mindfulness is always there to snap us right back to where we were and what we were doing and feeling. The best part about it is that we become better versions of ourselves without having to alter major things in our lives or how we are wired. Mindfulness accepts us as we are and helps us to transform at our own pace. You don't have to change your beliefs if you want to. You can hold unto the same beliefs and still practice and benefit from mindfulness.

"It sparks innovation. As we deal with our world's increasing complexity and uncertainty, mindfulness can lead us to effective, resilient, low-cost responses to seemingly intransigent problems."

8). Mindfulness is non judgemental

Mindfulness is not birthed by criticism and it should not be. Becoming judgemental and hard on ourselves about things does not give us the positive result of practicing mindfulness. When practicing mindfulness we are not to aim at suppressing or stopping our thoughts. Our goal should simply be to pay attention to our experiences as they arise without judging or labelling them in any way.

Mindfulness then allows us to become the watcher of sense perceptions, thoughts and emotions as they arise without getting caught up in them and being swept away in their current. As watchers, we are less likely to mechanically play out old habitual ways of thinking and living. It conjures an access to new freedom and choice in our lives.

"Mindfulness is about observation without criticism; being compassionate with yourself" (What Is Mindfulness?," n.d.).

The History and Origin of Mindfulness

Mindfulness practices have been around for a very long time. Mindfulness is derived from sati, a significant element of Buddhist tradition, and based on Zen, Vipassanā, and Tibetan meditation techniques. Some of the key individuals who have contributed to the popularity of mindfulness in the modern Western context include Thích Nhất Hạnh, Herbert Benson, Jon Kabat-Zinn, and Richard J. Davidson.

Among these individuals, the most recognised expert that substantially contributed to the concept of mindfulness is Jon Kabat-Zinn. Forty years ago, Jon Kabat-Zinn embraced the Buddhist contemplation practices and refined it for a secular age. Part of his works that gained popularity include: the popular book called 'Full Living Catastrophe' and an MBSR (Mindfulness-Based Stress Reduction) program. His works have been adopted in different places over the years: schools, hospitals, prisons, and other places. It has also been useful for mindfulness guides such as healthy aging, weight management, athletic performance, helping children with special needs, and as an intervention during the perinatal period.

Today, Mindfulness is gaining more popularity as a daily practice apart from Buddhist insight meditation and its application in clinical psychology. Mindfulness is being taught in educational institutions, side by side with endorsed mindfulness-related programs .

The difference betweenMindfulness and Mediation

The extent to which Mindfulness and Mediation contrast in meaning might seem obvious, but it is not. Most of the time, we tend to mistake one for the other, and then we intertwine them together blindly.

Here's the thing. Do not confuse mindfulness for a temporary state of mind that appears when we meditate and then vanishes shortly after. It is a continuous process that we step back into the present moment at any pont in time. Mindfulness may not totally take away stress, our challenges it other difficulties, but it helps us become more aware of unpleasant thoughts and feelings that arise and how we can handle them at the moment. We become thoughtful to respond, and cautious of how we express our anger and every other unpleasant emotion. It is used as a therapeutic technique.

Meditation on the other hand, lays the foundation for learning mindfulness. At first, we meditate to take charge of our her and now for a short period of time. As time goes on, we develop and then build our ability to take charge of present moments daily.

HOW CAN MINDFULNESS HELP YOU?

What can mindfulness do for you? What are the benefits of practicing mindfulness? Why should we practice it?

Studies have shown that practicing mindfulness, even for just a few weeks, can bring a variety of physical, psychological, and social benefits. Here are some of these benefits:

~ OUR BODY AND MIND

Mindfulness improves our bodies and minds. Practicing mindfulness meditation:

- boosts our immune system's ability to fight off illness
- improves sleep quality
- increases our intelligence
- creates clearer, more focused thinking and improves our mind's efficiency. It empowers our minds.

~ FOCUS

Mindfulness helps us focus. Researches show that mindfulness helps us tune out distractions and improves our memory, attention skills, and decision-making. More so, it enhances our visual attention processing. When we practice mindfulness meditation, we tend to display greater attentional functioning through the ability to show selective attention, better concentration and more.

A decent number of findings have proved that systematic mindfulness meditation training stimulates improvements in attention, awareness, and emotion (Treadway & Lazar, 2009).

~ MINDFULNESS AFFECTS THE WAY WE SEE OURSELVES

Mindful people tend to have a stronger sense of self consciousness and seem to act more in line with their values. They may also have a healthier body image and more secure self-esteem.

~RESILIENCE

Mindfulness makes us more resilient. It has been evidenced that mindfulness training could help veterans facing post-traumatic stress disorder, police officers, women who suffered child abuse, and caregivers. It literally builds up more resilience in us to negative feedback

~MINDFULNESS SUPPRESSES COMBAT BIAS

Even a brief mindfulness training can reduce our implicit biases and the biased language we use. One way this works, researchers have found, is by attenuating the cognitive biases that contribute to prejudice.

~BUSINESS

Mindfulness can be useful for businesses. Mindfulness training could help make leaders more confident, improve creativity, reduce multitasking, and improve client satisfaction.

~MINDFULNESS IS GOOD FOR FAMILIES

Mindfulness can help parents and couples that intend to start a family. Studies suggest that it may reduce pregnancy-related anxiety, stress, and depression in expectant parents, and may even reduce the risk of premature births and developmental issues. Parents who practice mindful parenting report less stress, more positive parenting practices, and better relationships with their kids; their kids, in turn, are less susceptible to depression and anxiety, and have better social skills. Mindfulness training for families may lead to less-stressed parents who pay more attention to their kids.

Mindfulness may also be beneficial to teenagers and children. It helps teens reduce stress and depression and increase their self-compassion and happiness.

~MINDFULNESS HELPS HEALTH CARE PROFESSIONALS

Practicing mindfulness helps health care professionals cope with stress, connect with their patients, and improve their general quality of life. It also helps mental health professionals by reducing negative emotions and anxiety, and increasing their positive emotions and feelings of self-compassion.

~ MINDFULNESS HELPS PRISONS

Evidence suggests mindfulness reduces anger, hostility, and mood disturbances among prisoners by increasing their awareness of their thoughts and emotions, helping with their rehabilitation and reintegration.

~ ELIMINATES ANXIETY AND DEPRESSION

With mindfulness, there is less stress, less worry and less negativity. Rather than worrying about what has happened or might happen, when we are in the 'present', we deal with whatever is happening. A study suggests it may be as good as antidepressants in fighting depression and preventing relapse.

Mindfulness helps us cope with feelings of anxiety, and even depression.Mindfulness reduces levels of anxiety. Mindfulness reduces depression too, as clinical trials are showing that mindfulness is as effective as medication with no side effects.

~ MEMORY

-Mindfulness sharpens your memory and increases your focus and attention.Mindfulness practice has been empirically linked to enhanced working memory capacity.

Mindfulness changes our brains. Research has found that it increases density of gray matter in brain regions linked to learning, memory, emotion regulation, and empathy. It shrinks the the brain's "fight or flight" center, the amygdala. This primal region of the brain, associated with fear and emotion, is involved in the initiation of the body's response to stress. This is the part of the brain responsible for so many destructive emotions like fear, unhappiness and anger.

~ HEIGHTENED METACOGNITIVE AWARENESS

This describes being able to detach from one's own feelings and mental processes—to step back and perceive them as transient, momentary occurrences rather than 'who we are'. In the Buddhist sense, this would relate to 'knowing' and 'freeing' the mind.

~ HAPPINESS

The more mindful you are, the happier you are. Mindfulness can literally transform your entire world from the inside out. Try out mindfulness and and how it relates to your happiness. Who knows? You might just discover the most incredible and wonderful surprise. You would find out that everything you've been searching for 'out there' — feelings of fulfilment, peace and wholeness — have been within you all along.

You might be wondering how exactly mindfulness makes us happy. Through practice, we can learn to decenter from negative 'ways of being' and free our minds. When we are present and live mindfully, we get past the 'noise' in our heads and begin to experience life more deeply. We see that the small things we tend to ignore aren't small after all.

Whether the smell of freshly cut grass, a tree in bloom, the warmth of an embrace, or a smile /gesture of kindness from a strange. We notice and savour the sublime in the most ordinary moments of each day. We treasure the precious moments that make up our whole life. Mindfulness turns out to also be the single most important determining factor in whether or not you will be happy in your life.

~ OUR WELLBEING

Mindfulness improves our well being in the following ways:

a). It impacts our mental health:- Mindfulness-based therapy and interventions have been created to take a more structured approach to addressing mental health symptoms. Mindfulness practice allows us to step back and accept our own mental processes without judgment.

Mindfulness also reduces mentally-related compulsive and addictive tendencies.

b). It impacts our physical health :- There is also research that suggests mindfulness may have a role in managing physical pain. In short, mindfulness is very effective for pain management.

Mindfulness also reduces stress. It has been linked to lower stress levels. Mindfulness training has also been shown to work better than any diet for effective long-term weight loss. Mindfulness fights obesity. Practicing mindful eating encourages healthier eating habits, helps people lose weight, and helps them savor the food they do eat. Pregnant women who practice mindful eating gain less weight during pregnancy, and have healthier babies.

Mindfulness improves health and boosts immunity. In fact, mindfulness is shown to have beneficial effects on many serious illnesses such as cancer and heart disease.

Mindfulness also reduces insomnia, increases your sense of well being and reduces lethargy and increases energy both mentally and physically.

c). It improves our emotional health:- Mindfulness improves your emotional and social intelligence and develops your empathy and compassion. It is also shown to improve relationships. It regulates and expresses your emotions.

Mindfulness fosters compassion and altruism. Research suggests mindfulness training makes us more likely to help someone in need and increases activity in neural networks involved in understanding the suffering of others and regulating emotions. Evidence suggests it might boost self-compassion as well.

When it comes to the way we think and feel, being mindful of our emotions helps us to switch to more positive mindsets and work towards being a 'better'—or at least, a happier—person. Mindfulness builds confidence and emotional resilience. Being mindful can help us manage our emotions and feelings in stressful situations;

Several studies have found that mindfulness increases positive emotions while reducing negative emotions and stress too.

MINDFULNESS ENHANCES SCHOOLS

There's scientific evidence that teaching mindfulness in the classroom reduces behavior problems, aggression, and depression among students, and improves their happiness levels, self-regulation, and ability to pay attention. Scholars argued that the application of mindfulness practice enhances the goals of education in the 21st century, which include adapting to a rapidly changing world and being a caring and committed citizen.

Teachers trained in mindfulness also show lower blood pressure, less negative emotion and symptoms of depression, less distress and urgency, greater compassion and empathy, and more effective teaching.

RELATIONSHIPS

Psychological evidence suggests that being able to practice mindfulness can foster greater relationship satisfaction by increasing your ability to deal with stress when conflict arises (Barnes et al., 2007).

It also plays a role in helping us effectively communicate with one another about our feelings in romantic relationships, as well as in more general interpersonal situations (Dekeyser et al., 2008). Dekeyser and colleagues find this is related to the role of mindfulness in helping us to become more emotionally self-aware, empathetic, and less socially anxious.

So, in less scientific terms, we've already seen earlier on how mindfulness helps us stop responding so instinctively based on our emotions. When we look more closely at mindfulness practice in romantic relationships, we can also see how it helps us deal with the stress of conflicts and communicate better.

Research suggests mindfulness training makes couples more satisfied with their relationship, makes each partner feel more optimistic and relaxed, and makes them feel more accepting of and closer to one another. Mindful couples may also recover more quickly from conflict.

In terms of relationships, as we'll see in a short while, it has positive implications for how we communicate and relate to those around us.

Practicing mindfulness in relationships (as we'll see in a second) can help us listen better, appreciate others more, and get along at work;

Mindfulness practice in everyday life can lead us to really savor experiences with new perspectives. Nonetheless, all the studies have one thing in common. That is, to reap the benefits, you'll want to find a method of mindfulness practice that works for you. When we meditate it doesn't help to fixate on the benefits, but rather to just do the practice, and yet there are benefits or no one would do it. When we're mindful, we reduce stress, enhance performance, gain insight and aware ness through observing our own mind, and increase our attention to others' well-being. We start to see things as they really are (instead of how we imagine them to be through the filter of our story and habitual patterns), so can respond effectively and appreciate more

MINDFULNESS AS A LIFESTYLE

What is Mindfulness as a lifestyle? Mindfulness as a lifestyle mindfulness as a practice. What then is mindfulness as a practice?

Mindfulness as a practice can be defined as a way of paying attention in a particular way: on purpose, in the present moment, and nonjudgmentally. It can be described as bringing one's complete attention to the present experience on a moment-to-moment basis.

Mindfulness practice involves the process of developing the skill of bringing one's attention to whatever is happening in the present moment.

It is one thing to talk eloquently on the subject of mindfulness and it is another thing to actually practice mindfulness. You've heard about mindfulness a couple of times, and you've probably talked about it too. But, how about trying it? If you're trying it, how well do you walk your talk?

Infusing mindfulness in our day-to-day living requires practice. Without practice, we won't be able to live a life conscious of mindfulness. With that being said, how do we practice mindfulness as a lifestyle?

There are two major forms of mindfulness practice. They are; formal(meditation) and informal(non-meditation) practices. The formal practice of mindfulness is commonly known as meditation. Meditation is the practice of sustaining attention on body, breath or sensations, or whatever arises in each moment. Informal mindfulness is the application of mindful attention in everyday life. Studies have shown that meditation-based mindfulness practices can bring about physiological, psychological, and social benefits in our lives. It boosts the brain and alleviates physical ailments such as migraines and fibromyalgia. The benefits of mindfulness and meditation practice are almost more limitless. Meditation has generally have been touted for everyone. Meditators are best advice to start meditation within short periods of 10 minutes or so.

A meditation practice is typically done sitting, usually with eyes closed. You sit in a straight-backed chair or sit cross-legged on the floor or a cushion, close one's eyes and bring attention to either the sensations of breathing in the proximity of one's nostrils or to the movements of the abdomen when breathing in and out. Another method is one that can also be done lying down or even walking. For walking meditation, you focus on the movement of your body as you take step after step, your feet touching and leaving the ground—an everyday activity we usually take for granted. This exercise is often practiced walking back and forth along a path 10 paces long, though it can be practiced along most any path.

Other meditation practices also involve mantra (sound) or movement meditation. An example of such meditation is loving-kindness meditation, involves extending feelings of compassion toward people, starting with yourself then branching out to someone close to you, then to an acquaintance, then to someone giving you a hard time, then finally to all beings everywhere.

Informal practices are nonmeditation-based exercises that are specifically used in dialectical behavior therapy and in acceptance and commitment therapy. It is about living your life as if it really mattered, moment by moment. The informal practice simply involves doing things we are completely conscious of in our lives. It centers on how we apply mindfulness to the rest of our lives through mindfulness practices. The advantage of inducing informal practices means that we can practice mindfulness at the comfort of our home and at our own pace.

A simple guide you can follow to practice mindfulness in this form include:

- Taking up recommended exercises:- For a starting point, you could practice with easy videos and resources on mindfulness. You could also download a mindfulness app that would help you follow through.

- Turn your routines to mindfulness activities. E.g. washing the dishes, taking a walk. When you talk to people, listen to their views with a judgement-free. Instead of ending up with arguments, listen with the intention of peace and diplomacy so both of you can gain from each other. Also, speak publicly in a mindful manner. Do not let your emotions define you. Unwind them and see the impact. There are so many regular things you do that can be made into mindfulness practices. As long as you engage in this things fully mindful, you are practicing mindfulness.

Tips for practicing Mindfulness

- Make it an habit to always pay close attention to your breathing, especially when you feel intense emotions. Be aware of how you breathe in and out as your body rises and falls with every breath you take. Mindful breathing brings attention to the physical sensations of your breath as it flows in and out.

  Take a few moments to be aware of your breath. If you can feel your body relaxing as you take in and take out those breaths, then you're doing well.

- Whatever you do and wherever you go, focus only on the present. Focus on what goes on there and now. When you drift in thought, bring them back to the present, and pay more attention to what you're doing. Find these moments and reset your point of focus and purpose.

- Note whatever you're sensing or engaging in. If you are eating, notice on the taste, colour and every other detail of your food. Notice the sights, sounds, smells and feeling you sense all at once in your conscious awareness. Pay more attention by coming more aware of our own feelings and not reacting instinctively and paying greater attention to what others are saying.

- Relax and be in tune with your environment. Take sometime off from your buzz day and enjoy nature. Sometimes the best way to stay mindful is to put a hold to everything you're doing and just relax. Enjoy your existence.

- Recognize that your thoughts and emotions do not complete you. They should not be the pressure behind you nor the major force you need to take action. We must be able to control our mental process and our emotions all at once. We must be able to separate the negative thoughts and emotional patterns from the positive ones. You deserve to know your mind.

- Remember that being judgemental does not have to be part of you. Mindfulness practice means freeing your mind from things like this. It might be hard at first, but it becomes easier with time and effort. Treat things in ways that are judgement-free, including ourselves and people.

- Discover the activities that can tune you into your bodily sensations. Those activities could be opportunities to practice and experience more awareness pertaining to mindfulness. Make mindfulness part of your day and make it suit your radar. From driving to swimming, and to you hitting the shower.

- Be receptive. If we are more accepting of people and their views about things, we experience or anticipate less conflict. Being more accepting rather than resistant helps us increase our chances of a positive, even productive, response from others. In other words, we're more likely to come to a useful means of resolution, as others will usually be more accepting in turn.

  Allow yourself to be who you are, and permit others to do the same with your hospitality. Being accommodating can encourage greater self-expression and creativity. In the end, it all links right back to acceptance, which helps us all flourish as people.

- Appreciating others by valuing and fostering deeper relationships with your significant other, at the workplace,etc. Appreciating others births significant implications and benefits.

The thing about Mindfulness-practice is that all you have to do is to basically pick something that feels appealing and interesting to you, and don't be afraid to go for it.

If you want to go further by turning it into a skill, you can adopt these exercises or components used in John Kabat-Zinn's Mindfulness Based Stress Reduction Program (MBSR) for meditation-based practices:

- Mindful breathing. In this meditation practice, one does not try to control one's breathing, but attempts to simply be aware of one's natural breathing process/rhythm. When engaged in this practice, the mind will often run off to other thoughts and associations, and if this happens, you may notice that the mind has wandered. Yet, in an accepting, non-judgmental way, make effort to put your concentration back on breathing.

- Body Scan. This is technique where you being to attention every part of your body from head to toe. The attention is directed at various areas of the body and noting body sensations that happen in the present moment.

- The raisin exercise. This is where you slowly use all of your senses, one after another, to mindfully observe a raisin in great detail, from the way it feels in your hand to the way it tastes in your mouth. This exercise is intended to help you focus on the present moment, and can be tried with different foods.

  By enabling reconnection with internal hunger and satiety cues, mindful eating has been suggested to be a means of maintaining healthy and conscious eating patterns.

- Other approaches include practising yoga asanas while attending to movements and body sensations, and walking meditation.

While trying out these exercises, understand that there are several exercises designed to develop mindfulness meditation. Regardless, these different types of mindfulness practices have different benefits. It might take some experimentation to find the practice that's right for you.

UNDERSTANDING ANXIETY

To understand what anxiety is, we need to work through it by starting with the basics.

What is Anxiety?

Firstly, Anxiety is the feeling we get when we are worried, tensed or afraid about things that are about to happen or that could possibly happen later in future.

Secondly, Anxiety is also a natural response we humans exhibit when we are faced by an uncomfortable situation, like when we are under a threat, or we are about to have a job interview we're nervous about. This response is also known as the "fight, flight or freeze response", where we react to situations and find ways to adjust to unpleasant circumstances. As we adopt methods of reacting and adjusting to these situations, our bodies produce hormones that enables us to act faster and be more alert. Our heart beat faster, as blood pumps more to where it's needed the most.

When we feel like such threat or unpleasant situation has passed, our bodies produce other hormones that help us relax our muscles, and then the anxiety stops.

Lastly, Anxiety can be defined using the three levels of experience: physical, cognitive and emotional experience.

Physical experience are our bodily sensations, our ambience, feelings or mood. They could be hot, cold, tingly, tense, relaxed, achy, painful,etc.

Cognitive experiences are mental or intellectual phenomena or anything else that affects our thoughts or thinking. They are frequently expressed verbally, visually or imaginary. For instance, when we motivate ourselves with mantras like "You can do it Toby, you got this", or when we replay what we had for lunch earlier on or even what we hope to have for lunch.

Emotional experiences are the hardest to define, because they are versatile and they constitute both a minute of physical and cognitive experiences. E.g. when we feel that bodily sense of anger, there are thoughts that run through our minds cognitively. Emotional experiences leads us to experience subjective feelings after we interpret something cognitively.

What are the differences and relationships between Anxiety and other related concepts?

Fear

Fear is an emotion that usually arises as a response to a perceived threat or danger. You see red-colored drops of what seems like blood on the floor, and you immediately fear because you consider the possibility that it might be the blood of someone you care about. But as you look closer, you find out that it's merely oil paint on the floor, and then our fear subsides. Fear tends to be present-oriented, temporary in duration, and based on a reasonable evaluation of danger.

Anxiety on the other hand, tends to be imaginary, irrational, future-inclined, and prolonged. For instance, after seeing those stains of red oil paint, we may hesitate to attach ourselves with that color, probably by choosing to have white wine and not red or choosing a yellow top and not red, because the effect it had on us makes us cringe. Then, we start to imagine how dangerous it would be to attach ourselves with the color, red.

Panic

Panic is a sudden burst of intense anxiety that peaks within a few minutes and often subsides after some minutes. Panic is typically triggered by a catastrophic interpretation of symptoms associated with the fight or flight response. E.g. 'I think I might faint with the way my heart is pounding.'

When people have repeated panic attacks, it is often triggered by worrying about the fact that they might actually have a panic attack. In a sense, panic is more or less anxiety about anxiety.

Worry

Even though we casually use the term worried to describe how we feel emotionally, worry is a form of problem-solving that tends to be repetitive, fast, negative, and self-evaluative, but is generally unproductive or unhelpful. Worry is almost always the primary factor that sustains anxiety and stress or causes it to recur frequently. It is similar to but distinct from problem-solving or planning.

Terror, Dread, Angst, Nervousness, etc.

These are all emotional variations on fear or anxiety. Dread, for instance, is similar to anxiety but is often more vague and pervasive, more intense, though perhaps not as acute, and slightly more existential in nature.

Everyone has experienced anxiety one way or the other at some point before. Yet, we all express anxiety differently. Our usual, daily activities are affected by anxiety sometimes, mostly because they could be stress-induced. Other causes of anxiety could be an horrible incident like the loss of a loved one or one's job, an accident, etc. It is normal only to a certain extent. However, if it gets to an amount where it becomes too persistent, overwhelming, uncontrollable and excessive for a longer period of time, then it can be an anxiety disorder; and that is not healthy.

Anxiety disorders could impair the way we function as normal human beings. Anxiety disorders are really distressing to handle or cope with. Some of the common anxiety disorders today include:

1. Generalized Anxiety Disorder (GAD)

GAD is an unceasing anxiety stimulated by excessive worry about a variety of things like failing a test, not being able to sleep, what happens if you are the only one left in the world,etc. People with generalized anxiety are often described with the familiar name "the worried well". Symptoms of GAD get worse during stressful events.

People with generalized anxiety disorder worry endlessly over everyday issues—like health, money, or family problems—even if they realize there's little cause for concern. They startle easily, can't relax, and can't concentrate. They find it hard to fall asleep or stay asleep. They may get headaches, muscle aches, or unexplained pains. Symptoms often get worse during times of stress.

Generalized anxiety disorder may be hereditary, which means it runs in families. It usually begins at an earlier age and symptoms may manifest themselves more slowly than in most other anxiety disorders. Generalized anxiety has been known to be prevalent in more women than men worldwide.

2. Panic Disorder

A panic attack is a sudden surge of intense fear or anxiety that peaks within minutes and is typically characterized by sweating, rapid heart rate, chest tightness, feeling lightheaded, etc. A person has panic disorder when they experience repeated panic attacks with persistent anxiety about having future panic attacks or their consequences. Persistent anxiety creates fear, ,which in turn leads to panic attacks. But, not all people who has panic attacks have panic disorder.

3. Specific Phobia

Anxiety-related to a specific situation or object such as flying, snakes, confined spaces, etc. In other words, people are irrationally afraid that a specific thing or situation will lead to panic, not that the specific thing or situation itself is dangerous. True specific phobias are relatively rare. The much common sort of specifici phobia are panic disorders that are similar to a specific phobia.

4. Social Anxiety/Phobia

Social anxiety is anxiety in social situations, typically when a person is exposed to the real or imagined scrutiny or judgment of others. Often social anxiety manifests as excessive worry and concern about how others are perceive you, like if they make jest of you at your back or they judge you. Without treatment, social phobia can last for years or even a lifetime. People with social phobia worry for days or weeks before a social event. They're often embarrassed, self-conscious, and afraid of being judged. They find it hard to talk to others. They may blush, sweat, tremble, or feel sick to their stomach when around other people.

5. Obsessive-Compulsive Disorder (OCD)

OCD is defined as the repeated presence of obsessions, compulsions, or both. Obsessions are recurrent and intrusive thoughts, images, or urges that cause significant anxiety or distress (E.g.: imagining your house exploding because you forgot to turn off the stove) which the person attempts to suppress or ignore. Compulsions are repetitive behaviors or rituals that an individual performs in order to alleviate the anxiety associated with an obsession (E.g.: washing your hands seven times before drying them, counting the number of steps in every building you enter, etc.). The key idea with OCD is that people treat intrusive mental activity (an event) as something dangerous or bad because they assume that either they are responsible for it or that it means something (i.e. they treat it as though it is an action).

6. Post-Traumatic Stress Disorder (PTSD)

PTSD occurs when a person is exposed to an actual or threatened trauma (e.g. rape, murder, etc.). People become afraid of something in their environment triggering a memory of a traumatic event and the negative thoughts, feelings, and sensations that may go along with it. As a result, they become preoccupied with avoiding any kind of cue or trigger for their trauma. This avoidance can easily lead to isolation, depression, and substance abuse, not to mention higher levels of anxiety. It results in the persistent experiencing of:

Recurrent intrusive and distressing memories of the trauma

Avoidance of objects or situations associated with the trauma

Changes in thinking and mood associated with the trauma

Increased arousal (e.g. hypervigilance, increased startle response) following the trauma.

7. Separation Anxiety

Separation anxiety is a distress regarding separation from an attachment figure, usually a parent. It's generally seen in childhood (e.g. school refusal behaviors), but can also occur in adults (e.g. anxiety when a spouse leaves town for business).

So, till when does anxiety becomes abnormal? When does a normal anxiety turn to an anxiety disorder?

The difference between everyday anxiety and an anxiety disorder is that most of those feelings for the former are channeled positively, as they boost our morale and energy. In short, they turn out to be helpful because they help us focus in a good way. However, anxiety disorder is the complete opposite.

Anxiety reaches clinical levels when it interferes with one's everyday life negatively, thereby disabling them. Anxiety disorders are popularly diagnosed through "maladaptive beliefs". These maladaptive beliefs help you determine what type of anxiety disorder a person has.

Understanding Anxiety Disorders

Anxiety disorders increases the risk of you facing other medical problems such as heart disease, diabetes, substance abuse, and depression. Anxiety disorders are basically anything, but positive. The good part is that most anxiety disorders are naturally easy to treat and take care of. How do we handle our anxiety disorder or people with anxiety disorders? The key to tackling them is understanding them.

A). Educate yourself

An important way to start understanding these anxiety issues or disorders is by gaining self awareness. Learn how it affects you and your relationship with people. Use such knowledge to erase any possible strain on your relationships with your family, friends, colleagues or lover who's facing anxiety issues. Talk about it openly, honestly and directly with them. You can always look out for you, especially your mental health when you are self conscious of it. Self awareness gives you an edge; one of them being that you can easily spot anxiety symptoms before hand. As you educate yourself, you start to understand your body too. If you're learning in order to connect with people who face anxiety issues, acknowledge that anxiety is never what they wish for. Deal with them with patience.

B). Apply what you learn

After educating yourself, the next thing is to put it into practice. Preach what you learn. Always bear in mind that anxiety is not a weakness. Be intentional about how well you communicate about your anxiety. When you or anyone else experiences panic attacks or otherwise, try breathing slowly and deeply at that moment. They help calm the anxiety and even stop it at times too. Although, it takes a lot of practice, but it's worth it. Whenever you are at work or you are cooking dinner, and the anxiety sets in, tame it by inhaling and exhaling deeply, so as to reconnect with yourself.

You could also go out for walks, engage yourself, your family and your friends in a conversation about it if possible, do exercises, etc. The whole point is to intervene when you need it. Do not hesitate to reach out if you need help or if you feel alone. Seek professional help like therapy as much as possible. Do not shame anybody for it. Nobody deserves to be treated in such way. When they make progress or when you make progress with managing your anxiety, recognise it and celebrate it. It helps you appreciate yourself or that person more.

When you understand that anxiety is actually a mental health issue that is hard to manage, you would unconsciously think twice when you're dealing with people who have anxious thoughts. For instance, if your lover questions your fidelity, treat him or her patiently. It can be frustrating, but it would be really rewarding for both of you at the end, if you deal with it one on one. At the same time, know when to set boundaries about those anxious reactions and when to embrace them. If it gets over the top with them, let the know. Do not hold it in.

You could opt for counseling, in order to address it calmly. Practice coping skills for yourself or that person who needs it.

C). Be observant

For you to successfully manage an anxiety disorder that you have or someone close to you possesses, you need to be observant. Examine yourself or that person for any symptoms of anxiety disorders. On several occasions, these symptoms are not always obvious enough to discern, because they appear mostly in the trivial things we do. Examine meticulously how anxiety tends to define our personal choices, decisions and response to things. It could be our behaviour towards people, shopping habits, relationships, perfectionism or more.

Watch out for those anxiety symptoms; including shortness of breath, insomnia and anxiety attacks, stress or a fight-or-flight response. In other cases, they may be include getting angry too quickly, being easily irritable and controlling, being distracted and having trouble focusing, coming across as overly critical and exhibiting avoidant or passive aggressive behavior.

The activities in this book are designed to be apart of a self-improvement plan!

Mind Full vs Mindful- Explore the difference between mind full and mindful. Take a second to list moments and experiences that make you feel overwhelmed, sad or messy. Then make a list of moments and experiences that make them feel calm, nice and balanced like eating a warm, chocolate chip cookie.

1.) What are your thoughts about this activity?

2.) Do you feel that this activity was helpful? If so, why?

3.) After completing this activity, what did you learn about yourself?

4.) What emotions did you experience?

MIND FULL VS. MINDFUL

MIND FULL

Mind FULL is future focused. It adds two items to your to-do list for each one you check off. It is messy, sad and overwhelming.

MINDFUL

Mind FULL is future focused. It adds two items to your to-do list for each one you check off. It is messy, sad and overwhelming.

List the things that you think are Mind full or Mindful.

MIND FULL	MINDFUL

Jar of Thoughts- There are a hundreds of thoughts that enter your head daily from the time you wake up in the morning and with every interaction you have throughout the day. It's important for us to analyze the type of thoughts that we have; and monitor how long that we have those those. Make a list of their thoughts and identify what type of thought, (I need to improve my dance skills- neutral thought or I attract friends easily- positive thought). The lid being opened is a reflection of us having the ability to keep thoughts are lets thoughts go

1.) What are your thoughts about this activity?

_____
_____
_____
_____

2.) Do you feel that this activity was helpful? If so, why?

_____
_____
_____
_____

3.) After completing this activity, what did you learn about yourself?

_____
_____
_____
_____

4.) What emotions did you experience?

_____
_____
_____
_____

JAR OF THOUGHTS

When we can see our thoughts, we can better understand they are a passing moment in time.

Write own you current thoughts, either good or bad, in the jar below. The lid remains off so that the thoughts can come and go as they please.

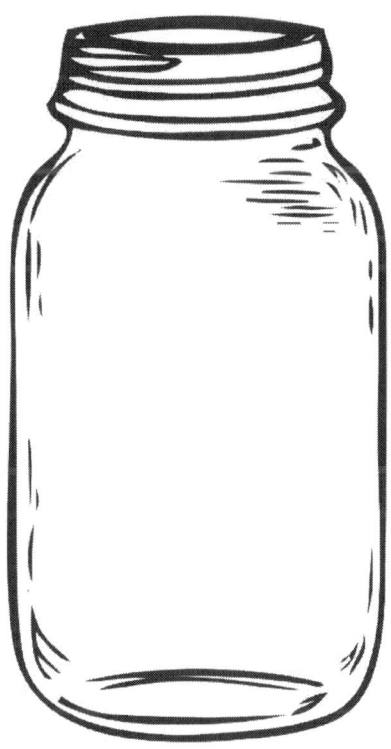

Mindful or Unmindful- There are times where we are mindful of our actions and words and sometimes we are unmindful of those same things. Categorize the mindful and the unmindful events on a chart and engage them in a discussion about their choices. Create a list of times when you are mindful or unmindful of your actions and words. Create an action plan to become more mindful.

1.) What are your thoughts about this activity?

_____
_____
_____
_____

2.) Do you feel that this activity was helpful? If so, why?

_____
_____
_____
_____

3.) After completing this activity, what did you learn about yourself?

_____
_____
_____
_____

4.) What emotions did you experience?

_____
_____
_____
_____

MINDFUL OR UNMINDFUL

Read and circle the mindful action below.

Practicing a new skill like music or sports until you feel that your body is improving.

Doing too many things at one time.

Thinking about an upcoming deadline while taking a walk.

Shout loudly when people are reading.

Leaving a belonging in a friend's house or in school.

Show kindness to someone who is scared or needy.

Train Your Brain- Introduce this activity by repeating the chant " I will become more aware of myself and my environment". Perform this 5 times and write down at least two thoughts that you remember directly after repeating the chant. We can train our brain to have positive thoughts by doing an exercise similar to this. Place the thoughts in the "what I should tell my brain and what I should not tell my brain" sections. Make a list of things that you tell yourself and write it in the chart. The goal is to focus on things that you should tell your brain.

1.) How did the children respond to this activity

_____
_____
_____

2.) Were there any children that didn't respond well to this activity? If so, why?

_____
_____
_____

3.) Which children responded really well to this activity? If so, why?

_____
_____
_____

4.) What emotions were experienced ?

_____
_____
_____

TRAIN YOUR BRAIN

Read the sentences below and write them in the given sections.

WHAT I SHOULD TELL MY BRAIN	WHAT I SHOULD NOT TELL MY BRAIN

- I cannot do this.
- I believe in myself.
- I am not capable enough.
- I will fail this test.
- I give up.
- I will find a way to do this.
- I will keep hard-working.

Mindfulness Word Search- Identify the top, three words that represent your personality traits with examples. Perform this exercise with a friend and share your thoughts.

1.) What are your thoughts about this activity?

_____

_____

_____

_____

2.) Do you feel that this activity was helpful? If so, why?

_____

_____

_____

_____

3.) After completing this activity, what did you learn about yourself?

_____

_____

_____

_____

4.) What emotions did you experience?

_____

_____

_____

_____

MINDFULLNESS WORD SEARCH

Search the words given below and encircle them.

```
G R A T I T U D E Q A P Y M M A I Q
A F T Y A B X O R F A A H L O G H U
C F O R G I V E I L H T K V T W A A
O A W A S A S T Y N A I U T I A T R
M K L T S A V I N G S E Z B V N Y T
P O E R C A L M F E R N S A A T M E
R P Y U B U Y F H A C C N T S D R
O L S S A C A T O S A E H J I A Q L
M T H T N V M A P Y F T X U O T M O
I R K U Y Y P E E N I A I Y N A N V
S E G F S A C R E A T I V I T Y M E
E O A L S N B K F I A B R E A T H E
```

CALM	CREATIVITY
GRATITUDE	COMPROMISE
TRUST	HOPE
PATIENCE	FORGIVE
LOVE	MOTIVATION
BREATHE	FAITH

Values Exercise- Begin by writing the word values and share some people, events or things that you value. Jot the people, events or things that you value and discuss with a friend. Complete the chart.

1.) What are your thoughts about this activity?

_____
_____
_____
_____

2.) Do you feel that this activity was helpful? If so, why?

_____
_____
_____
_____

3.) After completing this activity, what did you learn about yourself?

_____
_____
_____
_____

4.) What emotions did you experience?

_____
_____
_____
_____

VALUES EXERCISE

Determine your core values. From the list below, choose and write down at least 5 core values that resonates with you.

VALUES on which I am proud of myself	VALUES with which I don't associate myself	Values that I showed today	What should I keep doing?
Compassion	Bullying	Helped out a friend	Keep looking out for friends

Breathing Exercise- Take a moment to understand the way that you breathe affects your whole body. Breathing exercises are a good way to relax, reduce tension and relieve stress. These type of exercises supports mindfulness and reflection. With a friend open a discussion by asking, how did that make you feel? What were some of your thoughts during this process?

1.) What are your thoughts about this activity?

_____
_____
_____
_____

2.) Do you feel that this activity was helpful? If so, why?

_____
_____
_____
_____

3.) After completing this activity, what did you learn about yourself?

_____
_____
_____
_____

4.) What emotions did you experience?

_____
_____
_____
_____

BREATHING EXERCISE

Start with the top left corner of the polygon. Go towards the right and trace each part with your finger for 3 seconds while you breathe in and breathe out.

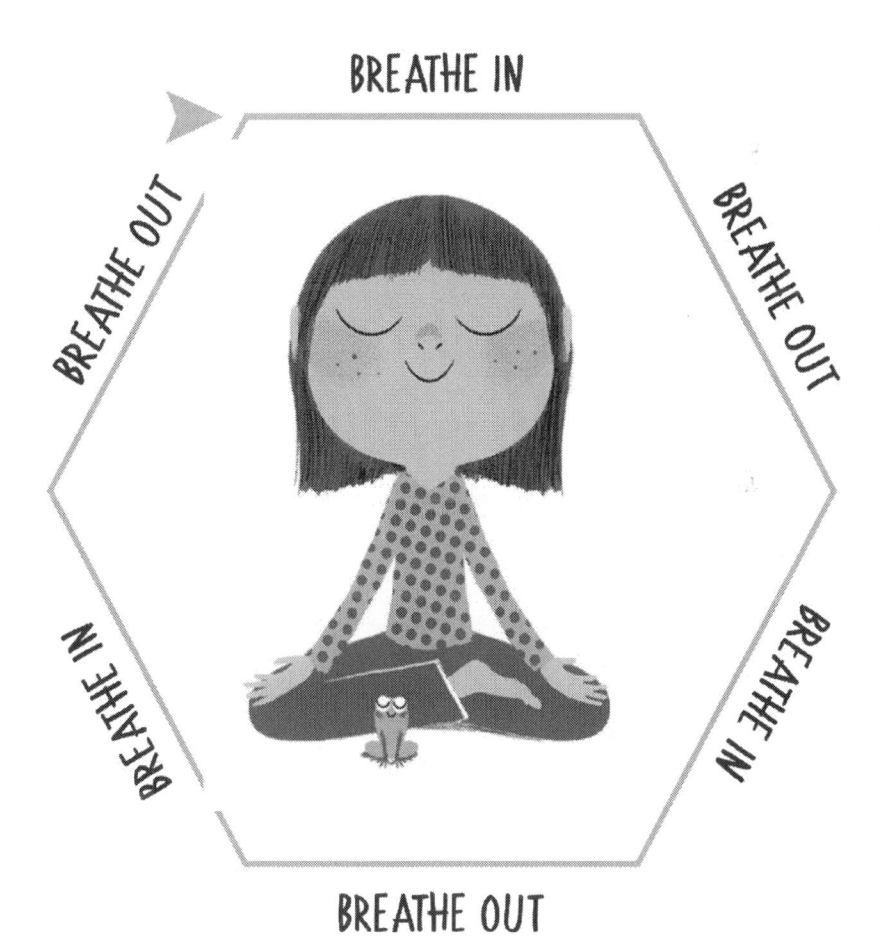

BREATHE IN

BREATHE OUT

BREATHE OUT

BREATHE IN

BREATHE IN

BREATHE OUT

Gratitude Chart- It's important to reflect on the good things in life. Reflecting on the good things in life can help keep you happy and healthy. (Being mindful of positive thoughts is great). Make a list of people, events or things that you are grateful for. Complete the chart. Place the chart in a location where it can be seen and reflected upon daily

1.) What are your thoughts about this activity?

_____
_____
_____
_____

2.) Do you feel that this activity was helpful? If so, why?

_____
_____
_____
_____

3.) After completing this activity, what did you learn about yourself?

_____
_____
_____
_____

4.) What emotions did you experience?

_____
_____
_____
_____

GRATITUDE CHART

Reflecting on the good things in life can also help keep you happy and healthy. You could keep a gratitude chart and fill it in every night. Think of something that makes you feel grateful.

I HAVE EXPRESSED MY GRATITUDE BY DOING THIS TODAY!

	MONDAY	TUESDAY	WEDNESDAY	THURSDAY	FRIDAY
I AM GRATEFUL FOR THIS PERSON TODAY					
I AM GRATEFUL FOR THIS THING HAPPENED TODAY					
I AM GRATEFUL FOR THIS EMOTION TODAY					
I AM EXPRESSED MY GRATITUDE BY DOING THIS TODAY					

Mindful Coloring- Mindful coloring ask us to focus on how we choose and apply color to in a design to bring awareness to the present moment. We feel more relaxed by paying attention to the present moment. Color the coloring page and write sentences that reflect how you felt while coloring.

1.) What are your thoughts about this activity?

_____
_____
_____
_____

2.) Do you feel that this activity was helpful? If so, why?

_____
_____
_____
_____

3.) After completing this activity, what did you learn about yourself?

_____
_____
_____
_____

4.) What emotions did you experience?

_____
_____
_____
_____

MINDFUL COLORING

"Mandala" is a Sanskrit word that means "circle" and represents how we are all connected and part of a wider universe. Colouring the mandala teaches kids patience and harmony, as well as provides a relaxing experience in which the kids can use colour to express themselves.

Color the Mandala given below.

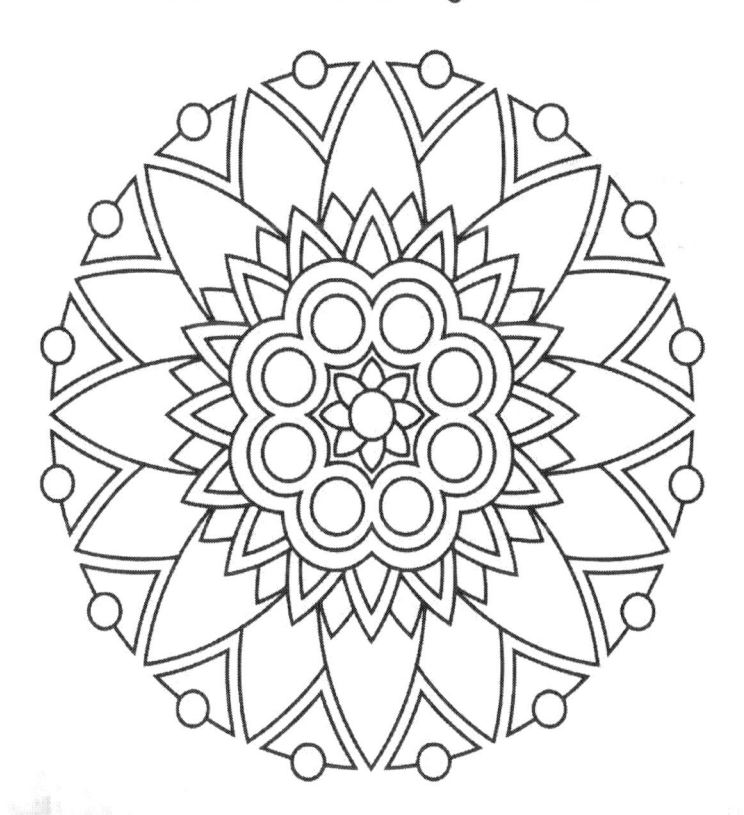

Weekly Goal Reflection- Introduce a quote relevant to mindfulness or awareness, "Mistakes are proof that you are trying" or "Our life is shaped by our minds, for we become what we think -Buddha". An important strategy to help you become mindful is setting goals around mindfulness and being aware of self. Complete the weekly goal reflection activity.

1.) What are your thoughts about this activity?

_____
_____
_____
_____

2.) Do you feel that this activity was helpful? If so, why?

_____
_____
_____
_____

3.) After completing this activity, what did you learn about yourself?

_____
_____
_____
_____

4.) What emotions did you experience?

_____
_____
_____
_____

WEEKLY GOAL REFLECTION

> A goal without a plan is just a wish...

Draw your weekly goal in the box and determine your weekly goal reflection below.

This week I did/ didn't make my goal. Why?

_____
_____
_____
_____
_____
_____

Overall, I would rate my efforts towards my goal.

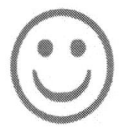

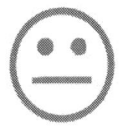

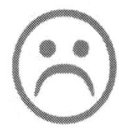

☺   😐   ☹

Mindful Weekly Challenge- Begin by stating "Mindfulness practice can help us to increase our ability to regulate emotions, decrease stress and anxiety". Show a chart, labeled at home or at work, and categorize the topics outlined on the chart. Take a second to notice how many ways that you can be mindful weekly.

1.) What are your thoughts about this activity?

_____
_____
_____
_____

2.) Do you feel that this activity was helpful? If so, why?

_____
_____
_____
_____

3.) After completing this activity, what did you learn about yourself?

_____
_____
_____
_____

4.) What emotions did you experience?

_____
_____
_____
_____

MINDFUL WEEKLY CHALLENGE

Let's see how many squares you can complete this week.

Read a book to a younger child.	Help your mom carry the groceries inside.	Share your food with your friend.
Write a nice letter to your teacher.	Say sorry for doing something wrong.	Give a nice compliment.
Acknowledge eveything that surrounds you.	Watch the sunrise.	Help someone before they ask.
Meditate for 5 minutes.	Express how you feel.	Notice 3 things you can hear.

Relax Your Body- Begin by closing your eyes and picture a place that makes you feel relaxed. Experiment with posture. Respond to the questions and reflect.

1.) What are your thoughts about this activity?

_____
_____
_____
_____

2.) Do you feel that this activity was helpful? If so, why?

_____
_____
_____
_____

3.) After completing this activity, what did you learn about yourself?

_____
_____
_____
_____

4.) What emotions did you experience?

_____
_____
_____
_____

RELAX YOUR BODY

Perform the activity and answer the questions below.

ACTIVITY

We are now going to experiment with our posture — the way we are sitting.

Try leaning from side to side, forward and back, roll your necks, and experiment with different ways to hold your body, head, and shoulders until you find a comfortable, balanced way to sit.

What was the most comfortable way to sit?

How do you feel when your body is slouched over?

How do you feel when you are sitting up straight?

Slow Down Your Mind- Find pictures of people with different facial expressions. Distinguish your interpretations and emotions based off of the facial expressions. Share this activity with a friend.

1.) What are your thoughts about this activity?

_____
_____
_____
_____

2.) Do you feel that this activity was helpful? If so, why?

_____
_____
_____
_____

3.) After completing this activity, what did you learn about yourself?

_____
_____
_____
_____

4.) What emotions did you experience?

_____
_____
_____
_____

SLOW DOWN YOUR MIND

Take a moment to observe the picture and anwer the questions below.

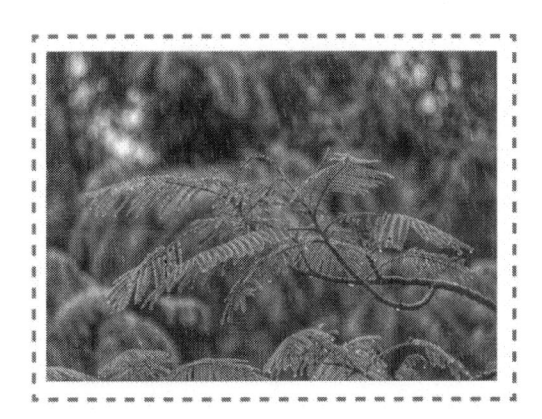

Just describe what you see in completely objective terms. Just notice colors, shapes, shades, etc. Write what you see here.
_____
_____
_____

Now notice the memories and thoughts that come up when you look at this picture. Allow your mind to wander as it will,   and write down what "pops" into your mind as it comes up. Take 1-2 minutes to do this.
_____
_____
_____
_____

Mindful Listening

1.) What are your thoughts about this activity?

2.) Do you feel that this activity was helpful? If so, why?

3.) After completing this activity, what did you learn about yourself?

4.) What emotions did you experience?

MINDFUL LISTENING

An owl can hear sounds that are close up and far away, and can also be silent when needed.

Go on a "sound hunt" as an owl. What do you hear close up? What do you hear far away? Write and draw your observations.

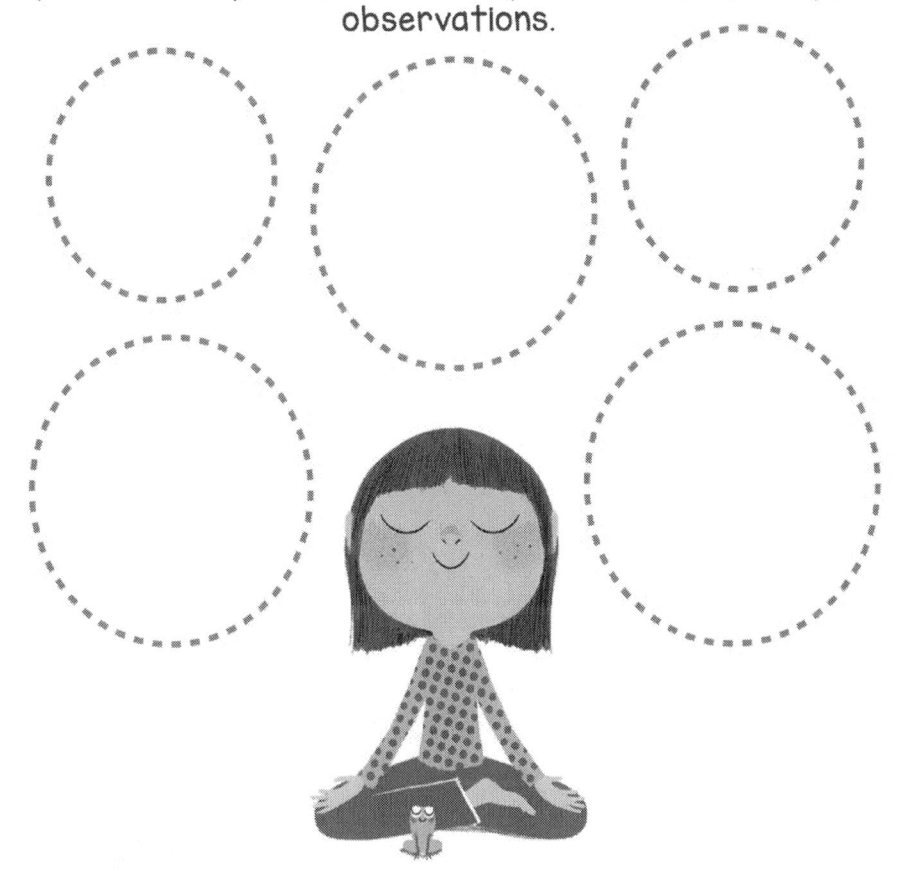

The Present Moment- Begin by looking at photographs of past, present and future communities, ex. Show pictures of Chicago in the past, present and future expectations of Chicago's community. Write down positive moments and experiences that have taken place in your lives and dissect how it made you feel.

1.) What are your thoughts about this activity?

_____
_____
_____
_____

2.) Do you feel that this activity was helpful? If so, why?

_____
_____
_____
_____

3.) After completing this activity, what did you learn about yourself?

_____
_____
_____
_____

4.) What emotions did you experience?

_____
_____
_____
_____

THE PRESENT MOMENT

What is the difference between the past, the present, and the future? Below, write and/or draw about something that took place in the past, something that might take place in the future, and something that is happening right now.

PRESENT

PAST

FUTURE

Beauty Inside Me- Everyone has a good inside of them. Discuss some good things that you have done. Even if you make bad choice or someone who is deemed bad, still have some good in them. List five things that make you beautiful.

1.) What are your thoughts about this activity?

_____
_____
_____
_____

2.) Do you feel that this activity was helpful? If so, why?

_____
_____
_____
_____

3.) After completing this activity, what did you learn about yourself?

_____
_____
_____
_____

4.) What emotions did you experience?

_____
_____
_____
_____

BEAUTY INSIDE ME

Write down the things that make you beautiful.

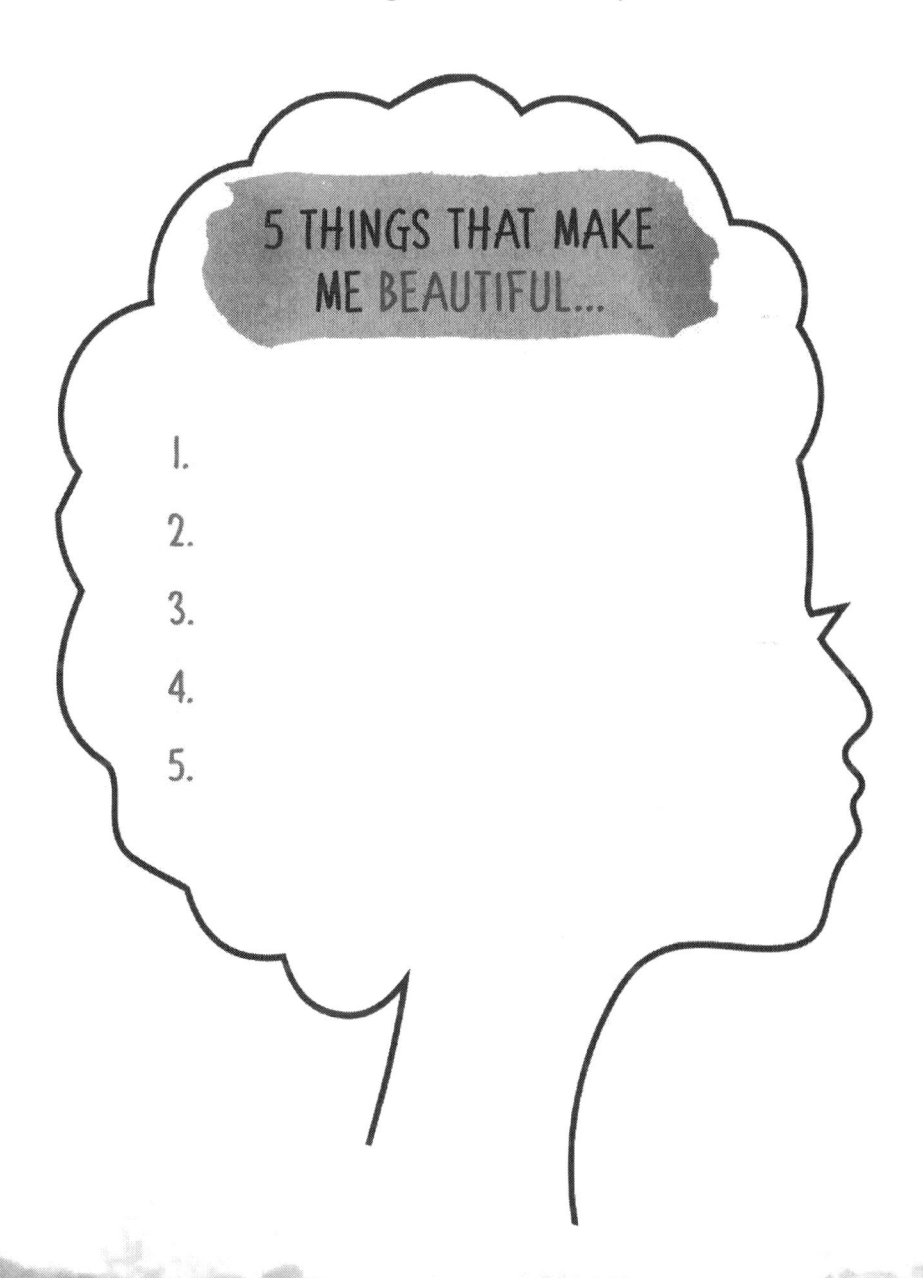

5 THINGS THAT MAKE ME BEAUTIFUL...

1.
2.
3.
4.
5.

Recognizing Emotions- Write the word emotion and explain what it mean to you. Emotion is the state of one's mood, circumstances, or relationships with others. Show the emotions with body language (happy, timid, happy, enthusiastic, solemn). It's clear that emotions are best when they are controlled. Draw faces for the specified emotion. Interpret what the drawing means to you.

1.) What are your thoughts about this activity?

_____
_____
_____
_____

2.) Do you feel that this activity was helpful? If so, why?

_____
_____
_____
_____

3.) After completing this activity, what did you learn about yourself?

_____
_____
_____
_____

4.) What emotions did you experience?

_____
_____
_____
_____

RECOGNIZING EMOTIONS

Draw the faces based on their emotions.

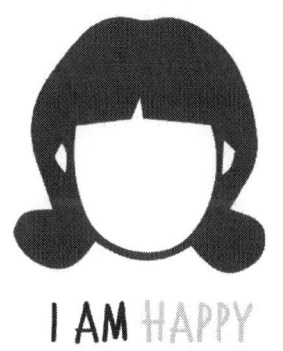

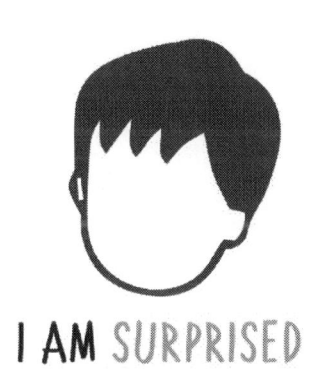

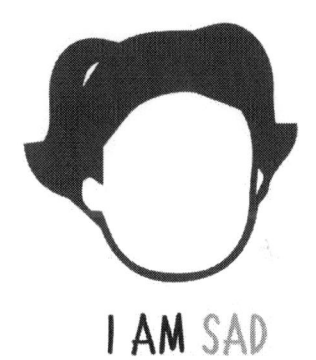

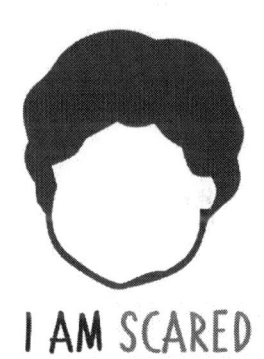

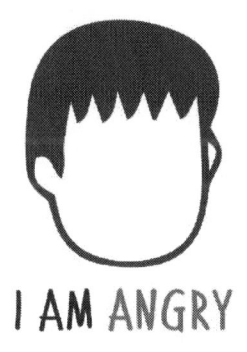

I AM HAPPY

I AM SAD

I AM SURPRISED

I AM SCARED

I AM ANGRY

Mindful Eating Exploration- Complete the handout and look at the importance of healthy eating and how specific vegetables, fruit and herbs increase positive body functions.

1.) What are your thoughts about this activity?

_____
_____
_____
_____

2.) Do you feel that this activity was helpful? If so, why?

_____
_____
_____
_____

3.) After completing this activity, what did you learn about yourself?

_____
_____
_____
_____

4.) What emotions did you experience?

_____
_____
_____
_____

MINDFUL EATING EXPLORATION

Draw the faces based on their emotions.

> Mindful eating is the practice of cultivating an open-minded awareness of how the food we choose to eat affects one's body, feelings, mind, and all that is around us.

What did you choose to eat?

How did it:

Look: _____

Smell: _____

Feel: _____

Taste: _____

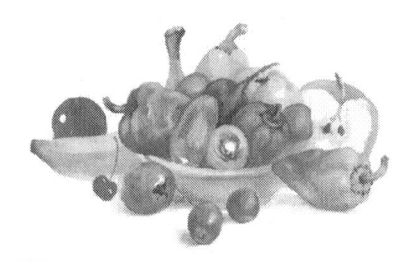

What Brings You Joy?- What is the meaning of joy? Create a list of things that bring you joy and happiness. Do this exercise with a friend and share with each other?

1.) What are your thoughts about this activity?

_____

_____

_____

_____

2.) Do you feel that this activity was helpful? If so, why?

_____

_____

_____

_____

3.) After completing this activity, what did you learn about yourself?

_____

_____

_____

_____

4.) What emotions did you experience?

_____

_____

_____

_____

WHAT BRINGS YOU JOY?

What are the things in your life that bring you the most joy? Use the space below to write or draw.

PEOPLE	PLACES
THINGS	EXPERIENCES

Mindful Yoga- Yoga is an exercise for mental, physical and spiritual health that support mindfulness. Look up simple yoga poses and engage in a few of them. Visualize positive images during poses. Play calming music. Reflect on how you feel and the thoughts that came to mind.

1.) What are your thoughts about this activity?

_____
_____
_____
_____

2.) Do you feel that this activity was helpful? If so, why?

_____
_____
_____
_____

3.) After completing this activity, what did you learn about yourself?

_____
_____
_____
_____

4.) What emotions did you experience?

_____
_____
_____
_____

WHAT BRINGS YOU JOY?

An exploration of what mindfulness is, its benefits and how can we bring it into our daily lives and our yoga practice.

Color the girl in yoga position.

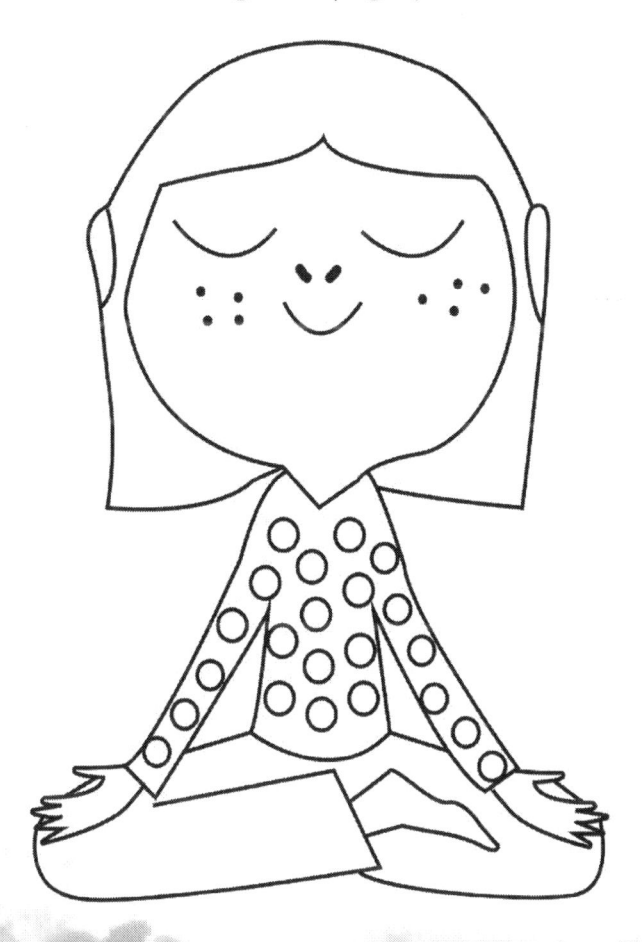

Made in the USA
Monee, IL
27 April 2020